MICROBIAL CODE FOR IMMEDIATE CONTROL OF MICROBIAL OUTBREAK

BY

RAHALI LAWALI

TABLE OF CONTENTS: *PAGE N0.*

INTRODUCTION

Although, **human** benefit symbiotically by the presence of **microbes** inside the body inform of normal flora, the violation of the ethics of the relationship most often by human produces a very serious damage on the later than on the former. The worst of such damages is recorded during an **outbreak** in which **bacteria** becomes the master minder .It excels other microbes; it is ready to engulfed human species whenever they trigger its outbreak. Bacteria have a code that gives it the honor to be the mother of all microbes.

BRIEF REVIEW OF MICROBIAL OUTBREAK

Cholera and Tuberculosis are among the major causes of outbreak among the human communities. They differ in their geographical interest; the former remained a daunting challenge among the developing countries, while the later is still producing medical alarm in the developed countries. The health implication of an outbreak can be summarized in the following ways:

-It causes rapid draining and shrinking of human resources and economy

-It attacks and disturbs human emotionally and socially.

WHO, CDC & other health agencies have taken into account the recent outbreaks caused by the above infectious diseases in various regions across the globe. We can arrest these microbial activities if we follow strictly the seven fundamentals for immediate control of microbial outbreak

MICROBIAL- CODE IN LINE WITH BACTERIAL SEGMENTED CODE:

Working From The First Dimension, We Have:

Input= [O^I x Q] A Slide per Letter

INPUT = BACTERIA

DATA

O -26

I - 10letters: 7,6,5, 4,3,2,1,0

Q-b= 1, a =0, c = 2, t = 19, e=4, r= 17, i=8, a=0

COMPUTING

b[26^7 x 1] + a[26^6 x 0] +c[26^5 x 2] + t[26^4 x 19] +e[26^3 x 4] +r[26^2 x 17] + i[26^1 x 8] + a[26^0 x 0]

OUTPUT IN FIGURES

[8064337476]-this is the Cardinal value of the word 'bacteria'

Hence, to derive ***Bacterial-Segmented Code***, each one of the definite digit inside the above cardinal values need to appear only once.

[8064337476]= **[8-6-4-3-7]-Bacterial -Segmented Code**

Interpretation Of Bacterial -Segmented Code

INPUT = ALGAE

COMPUTING

a[26^4 x 0] +l[26^3 x 11] +g[26^2 x 6] + a[26^1 x 0] + e[26^0 x 4]

OUTPUT

[197396]

[35]

[**8**]= [**8**-6-4-3-7]

It implies that algae are one of the major classes of microbes.

INPUT = VIRUSES

COMPUTING

v[26^6 x 21] +i[26^5 x 8] + r[26^4 x 17] +u[26^3 x 20] +s[26^2 x 18] + e[26^1 x 4] + s[26^0 x 18]

OUTPUT

[6590414706]

[42]

[**6**]- [8-**6**-4-3-7]

It implies that viruses are one of the major classes of microbes.

INPUT = FUNGUS

COMPUTING

f[26^5 x 5] + u[26^4 x 20] +n[26^3 x 13] +g[26^2 x 6] + u[26^1 x 20] + s[26^0 x 18]

OUTPUT

[68779482]

[51]

[**6**]- [8-**6**-4-3-7]

It implies that fungus is one of the major classes of microbes.

INPUT = PROTOZOA

DATA

O -26

I - 8letters: 7,6,5, 4,3,2,1,0

Q-p= 15, r =17, o = 14, t = 19, o=14, z= 25, o=14, a=0

COMPUTING

p[26^7 x 15] + r[26^6 x 17] +o[26^5 x 14] + t[26^4 x 19] +o[26^3 x14] +z[26^2 x 25] + o[26^1 x 14] + a[26^0 x 0]

OUTPUT

[125904005968]

[49]

[13]

[4]- [8-6-4-3-7]

It implies that protozoa are one of the major classes of microbes.

INPUT = BACTERIA

DATA

O -26

I - 8letters: 7,6,5, 4,3,2,1,0

Q-b= 1, a =0, c = 2, t = 19, e=4, r= 17, i=8, a=0

COMPUTING

b[26^7 x 1] + a[26^6 x 0] +c[26^5 x 2] + t[26^4 x 19] +e[26^3 x 4] +r[26^2 x 17] + i[26^1 x 8] + a[26^0 x 0]

OUTPUT

[8064337476]

[48]

[12]

[<u>**3**</u>]- [8-6-4-<u>**3**</u>-7]

It implies that Bacteria are one of the major classes of microbes.

INPUT =PROTISTS

DATA

O -26

I - 8letters: 7,6,5, 4,3,2,1,0

Q-p= 15, r =17, o = 14, t = 19, i=8, s= 18, t=19, s=18

COMPUTING

p[26^7 x 15] + r[26^6 x 17] +o[26^5 x 14] + t[26^4 x 19] +i[26^3 x 8] +s[26^2 x 18] + t[26^1 x 19] + s[26^0 x 18]

OUTPUT

[125903895928]

[61]

[<u>7</u>]- [8-6-4-3-<u>7</u>]

It implies that protists are one of the major classes of microbes.

Hence, Only Six Major Classes Of Microbes Were Realized In Line With Bacterial Segmented Code, Namely:

I-Algae

Ii-Viruses

Iii-Fungus

Iv-Protozoa

V-Bacteria

Vi-Protists

MICROBIAL PROXIMITY

Microbial Proximity Is Based On Number 3 & ?:

Working From The First Dimension, We Have:

Input= $[O^I \times Q]$ A Slide per Letter

INPUT = MICROBES

DATA

O -26

I - 8letters: 7,6,5, 4,3,2,1,0

Q-m= 12, i =8, c = 2, r = 17, o=14, b= 1, e=4, s=18

COMPUTING

$m[26^7 \times 12] + i[26^6 \times 8] + c[26^5 \times 2] + r[26^4 \times 17] + o[26^3 \times 14] + b[26^2 \times 1] + e[26^1 \times 4] + s[26^0 \times 18]$

OUTPUT

[98884826526]

[66]

[12]

[3]=?

INPUT = BACTERIA

DATA

O -26

I - 8letters: 7,6,5, 4,3,2,1,0

Q-b= 1, a =0, c = 2, t = 19, e=4, r= 17, i=8, a=0

COMPUTING

b[26^7 x 1] + a[26^6 x 0] +c[26^5 x 2] + t[26^4 x 19] +e[26^3 x 4] +r[26^2 x 17] + i[26^1 x 8] + a[26^0 x 0]

OUTPUT

[8064337476]

[48]

[12]

[3]=?

INPUT = HUMAN

DATA

O -26

I - 5letters: 4,3,2,1,0

Q-h= 7, u =20, m= 12, a= 0, n=13

COMPUTING

h[26^4 x 7] +u[26^3 x 20] + m[26^2 x 12] + a[26^1 x 0] + n[26^0 x 13]

OUTPUT

[3558477]

[39]

[12]

[3]=?

INPUT = OUTBREAK

DATA

O -26

I - 8letters: 7,6,5, 4,3,2,1,0

Q-o= 14, u =20, t = 19, b = 1, r=17, e= 4, a=0, k=10

COMPUTING

o[26^7 x 14] + u[26^6 x 20] +t[26^5 x 19] + b[26^4 x 1] +r[26^3 x 17] +e[26^2 x 4] + a[26^1 x 0] + k[26^0 x 10]

OUTPUT

[118850162610]

[39]

[12]

[3]=???---

INPUT = CHOLERA

DATA

O -26

I - 7letters: 6,5, 4,3,2,1,0

Q-c= 2, h =7, o = 14, l= 11, e=4, r= 17, a=0,

COMPUTING

c[26^6 x 2] +h[26^5 x 7] + o[26^4 x 14] +l[26^3 x 11] +e[26^2 x 4] + r[26^1 x 17] + a[26^0 x 0]

OUTPUT

[707595330]

[39]

[12]

[3] –*Hence, Cholera May be Among The Major Causes Of Outbreak*

INPUT =ANTHRAX

DATA

O -26

I - 7letters: 6,5, 4,3,2,1,0

Q-a= 0, n =13, t = 19, h= 7, r=17, a= 0, x=23

COMPUTING

a[26^6 x 0] +n[26^5 x 13] + t[26^4 x 19] +h[26^3 x 7] +r[26^2 x 17] +

a[26^1 x 0] + x[26^0 x 23]

OUTPUT

[163274979]

[48]

[12]

[3] –*Hence, Anthrax May be Among The Major Causes Of Outbreak*

INPUT =TUBERCULOSIS

DATA

O -26

I - 12letters: 11, 10, 9, 8, 7, 6,5, 4,3,2,1,0

Q-t= 19, u =20, b= 1, e= 4, c=2, u= 20, l=11 ,c= 2, l =11, o= 14, s= 18, i=8, s= 18

COMPUTING

t[26^{11} x 19]+u[26^{10} x20]+ b[26^9 x 1] + e[26^8 x 4] + r[26^7 x 17] +

$c[26^6 \times 2] + u[26^5 \times 20] + l[26^4 \times 11] + o[26^3 \times 14] + s[26^2 \times 18] + i[26^1 \times 8] + s[26^0 \times 18]$

OUTPUT

[72566289379289802]

[93]

[12]

[3] –*Hence, Tuberculosis May be Among The Major Causes Of Outbreak. Etc*

THE FUNDAMENTALS FOR IMMEDIATE CONTROL OF MICROBIAL OUTBREAK

Working From The First Dimension, We Have:

Input= $[O^I \text{ x } Q]$ A Slide per Letter

INPUT = OUTBREAK

DATA

O -26

I - 8letters: 7,6,5, 4,3,2,1,0

Q-o= 14, u =20, t = 19, b = 1, r=17, e= 4, a=0, k=10

COMPUTING

$o[26^7 \text{ x } 14] + u[26^6 \text{ x } 20] + t[26^5 \text{ x } 19] + b[26^4 \text{ x } 1] + r[26^3 \text{ x } 17]$

$+e[26^2 \text{ x } 4] + a[26^1 \text{ x } 0] + k[26^0 \text{ x } 10]$

OUTPUT

[118850162610]

Hence, to derive an ***Outbreak-Segmented Code***, each one of the definite digit inside the above cardinal values need to appear only once.

[118850162610] = **[1-8-5-6-2]- Outbreak -Segmented Code**

Interpretation Of An Outbreak -Segmented Code

INPUT = DRINKING

COMPUTING

$d[26^7 \text{ x } 3] + r[26^6 \text{ x } 17] + i[26^5 \text{ x } 8] + n[26^4 \text{ x } 13] + k[26^3 \text{ x } 10]$

$+i[26^2 \text{ x } 8] + n[26^1 \text{ x } 13] + g[26^0 \text{ x } 6]$

OUTPUT

[29448171928]

[55]

[10]

[**1**]- [**1**-8-5-6-2]

It implies that provision of portable "drinking" water is among the key fundamentals for the control of microbial outbreak

INPUT =BREATHING

COMPUTING

$b[26^8 \times 4] + r[26^7 \times 17] + e[26^6 \times 4] + a[26^5 \times 0] + t[26^4 \times 19] + h[26^3 \times 7] + i[26^2 \times 8] + n[26^1 \times 13] + g[26^0 \times 6]$

OUTPUT

[346612312000]

[28]

[10]

[**1**]- [**1**-8-5-6-2]

It implies that provision of adequate ventilation for "breathing" is among the key fundamentals for the control of microbial outbreak.

INPUT =DIRECT CONTACT

COMPUTING

$d[26^5 \times 3] + i[26^4 \times 8] + r[26^3 \times 17] + e[26^2 \times 4] + c[26^1 \times 2] + t[26^0 \times 19]$/+/ $c[26^6 \times 2] + o[26^5 \times 14] + n[26^4 \times 13] + t[26^3 \times 19] + a[26^2 \times 0] + c[26^1 \times 2] + t[26^0 \times 19]$

OUTPUT

[39601503]+[790445519]

[830047022]

[26]

[**8**]- [1-**8**-5-6-2]

It implies that avoiding "direct contact" is among the key

fundamentals for the control of microbial outbreak.

INPUT =OVERCROWDING

COMPUTING

o[26^{11} x 14] +v[26^{10} x 21] + e[26^{9} x 4] + r[26^{8} x 17]+c[26^{7} x 2] +r[26^{6} x 17] + o[26^{5} x 14] +w[26^{4} x 22] +d[26^{3} x 3] + i[26^{2} x 8] + n[26^{1} x 13]+ g[26^{0} x6]

OUTPUT

[54371071332908960]

[68]

[14]

[**5**]- [1-8-**5**-6-2]

It implies that avoiding "overcrowding" is among the key

fundamentals for the control of microbial outbreak

INPUT =FOOD INTAKE

COMPUTING

f[26^{3} x 5] +o[26^{2} x 14] + o[26^{1} x 14] + d[26^{0} x 3]/+/ i[26^{5} x 8] + n[26^{4} x 13] +t[26^{3} x 19] +a[26^{2} x 0] + k[26^{1} x 10] + e[26^{0} x 4]

OUTPUT

[97711]+[101325904]

[101423615]

[23]

[<u>**5**</u>]- [1-8-<u>**5**</u>-6-2]

It implies that supervision of "food intake" is among the key fundamentals for the control of microbial outbreak.

INPUT =BARRIER NURSING

COMPUTING

b[26^6 x 1] + a[26^5 x o] +r[26^4 x 17] +r[26^3 x 17] + i[26^2 x 8] + e[26^1 x 4]+ r[26^0 x17] /+/n[26^6 x 13] + u[26^5 x 20] +r[26^4 x 17] +s[26^3 x 18] + i[26^2 x 8] + n[26^1 x 13]+ g[26^0 x6]

OUTPUT

[316988689]+[4261623320]

[4578612009]

[42]

[<u>**6**</u>]- [1-8-5-<u>**6**</u>-2]

It implies that providing "barrier nursing" is among the key fundamentals for the control of microbial outbreak

INPUT =TRAVELLERS

COMPUTING

t[26^9 x 19] + r[26^8 x 17] + a[26^7 x 0] + v[26^6 x 21] +e[26^5 x 4] + l[26^4 x 11] +l[26^3 x 11] +e[26^2 x 4] + r[26^1 x 17] + s[26^0 x 18]

OUTPUT

[106717169978372]

[74]

[11]

[<u>**2**</u>]- [1-8-5-6-<u>**2**</u>]

It implies that restriction of movement of "travellers" is among the key fundamentals for the control of microbial outbreak.

Hence, the seven fundamentals for immediate control of microbial outbreak can be summarized as follow:

i-Provision Of Portable "Drinking" Water

ii- Provision Of Adequate Ventilation For "Breathing"

iii- Avoiding "Direct Contact"

iv- Avoiding "Overcrowding"

v- Supervision Of "Food Intake"

vi- Providing "Barrier Nursing"

vii- Restriction Of Movement Of "Travellers"

BRIEF HIGHLIGHTS ON THE DIGITAL VIEW OF THE FUNDAMENTALS FOR IMMEDIATE CONTROL OF MICROBIAL OUTBREAK.

MICROBES
microorganism, or microbe,[a] is a microscopic organism, which may exist in its single-celled form or in a colony of cells. The possible existence of unseen microbial life was suspected from ancient times, such as in Jain scriptures from 6th century BC India and the 1st century BC book On Agriculture by Marcus Terentius Varro. Microbiology, the scientific study of microorganisms, began with their observation under the microscope in the 1670s by Antonie van Leeuwenhoek. In the 1850s, Louis Pasteur found that microorganisms caused food spoilage, debunking the theory of spontaneous generation. In the 1880s, Robert Koch discovered that microorganisms caused the diseases tuberculosis, cholera and anthrax. Microorganisms include all unicellular organisms and so are extremely diverse. Of the three domains of life identified by Carl Woese, all of the Archaea and Bacteria are microorganisms. These were previously grouped together in the two domain system as Prokaryotes, the other being the eukaryotes. The third domain Eukaryota includes all multicellular organisms and many unicellular

protists and protozoans. Some protists are related to animals and some to green plants. Many of the multicellular organisms are microscopic, namely micro-animals, some fungi and some algae, but these are not discussed here.
They live in almost every habitat from the poles to the equator, deserts, geysers, rocks and the deep sea. Some are adapted to extremes such as very hot or very cold conditions, others to high pressure and a few such as Deinococcus radiodurans to high radiation environments. Microorganisms also make up the microbiota found in and on all multicellular organisms. A December 2017 report stated that 3.45-billion-year-old Australian rocks once contained microorganisms, the earliest direct evidence of life on Earth.[1][2]
Microbes are important in human culture and health in many ways, serving to ferment foods, treat sewage, produce fuel, enzymes and other bioactive compounds. They are essential tools in biology as model organisms and have been put to use in biological warfare and bioterrorism. They are a vital component of fertile soils. In the human body microorganisms make up the human microbiota including the essential gut flora. They are the pathogens responsible for many infectious diseases and as such are the target of hygiene measures.

RELATED SOURCE

https://en.wikipedia.org/wiki/Microorganism

PROVISION OF PORTABLE "DRINKING" WATER
Prevention and control of cholera outbreaks: WHO policy and recommendations *Prevention* *Measures for the prevention of cholera mostly consist of providing clean water and proper sanitation to populations who do not yet have access to basic services. Health education and good food hygiene are equally important. Communities should be reminded of basic hygienic behaviours, including the necessity of systematic hand-washing with soap after defecation and before handling food or eating, as well as safe preparation and conservation of food. Appropriate media, such as radio, television or newspapers should be involved in disseminating health education messages. Community and religious leaders should also be associated to social mobilization campaigns.* *In addition, strengthening surveillance and early warning greatly helps in detecting the first cases and put in place control measures. Conversely, routine treatment of a community with antibiotics, or mass chemoprophylaxis, has no effect on the spread of cholera, can have adverse effects by increasing antimicrobial resistance and provides a false sense of security.* *Key messages* *Provision of safe water, proper sanitation, and food safety are critical for preventing occurrence of cholera.* *Health education aims at communities adopting preventive behaviour for averting contamination.* ***RELATED SOURCE***

https://www.who.int/cholera/technical/prevention/control/en/index2.html

PROVISION OF ADEQUATE VENTILATION FOR "BREATHING"

Abstract

Background

Institutional transmission of airborne infections such as tuberculosis (TB) is an important public health problem, especially in resource-limited settings where protective measures such as negative-pressure isolation rooms are difficult to implement. Natural ventilation may offer a low-cost alternative. Our objective was to investigate the rates, determinants, and effects of natural ventilation in health care settings.

Methods and Findings

The study was carried out in eight hospitals in Lima, Peru; five were hospitals of "old-fashioned" design built pre-1950, and three of "modern" design, built 1970–1990. In these hospitals 70 naturally ventilated clinical rooms where infectious patients are likely to be encountered were studied. These included respiratory isolation rooms, TB wards, respiratory wards, general medical wards, outpatient consulting rooms, waiting rooms, and emergency departments. These rooms were compared with 12 mechanically ventilated negative-pressure respiratory isolation rooms built post-2000. Ventilation was measured using a carbon dioxide tracer gas technique in 368 experiments. Architectural and environmental variables were measured. For each experiment, *infection risk was estimated for TB exposure using the Wells-Riley model of airborne infection. We found that opening windows and doors provided median ventilation of 28 air changes/hour (ACH), more than double that of mechanically ventilated negative-pressure rooms ventilated at the 12 ACH recommended for high-risk areas, and 18 times that with windows and doors closed ($p < 0.001$). Facilities built more than 50 years ago, characterised by large windows and high ceilings, had greater ventilation than modern naturally ventilated rooms (40 versus 17 ACH; $p < 0.001$). Even within the lowest quartile of wind speeds, natural ventilation exceeded mechanical ($p < 0.001$). The Wells-Riley airborne infection model predicted that in mechanically ventilated rooms 39% of susceptible individuals would become infected following 24 h of exposure to untreated TB patients of infectiousness characterised in a well-documented outbreak. This infection rate compared with 33% in modern and 11% in pre-1950 naturally ventilated facilities with windows and doors open.*

Conclusions

Opening windows and doors maximises natural ventilation so that the risk of airborne contagion is much lower than with costly, maintenance-requiring mechanical ventilation systems. Old-fashioned clinical areas with high ceilings and large windows provide greatest protection. Natural ventilation costs little and is maintenance free, and is particularly suited to limited-resource settings and tropical climates, where the burden of TB and institutional TB transmission is highest. In settings where respiratory isolation is difficult and climate permits, windows and doors should be opened to reduce the risk of airborne contagion.

RELATED SOURCE

https://journals.plos.org/plosmedicine/article?id=10.1371/journal.pmed.0040068

AVOIDING "DIRECT CONTACT"

Diseases that can be transmitted by direct contact are called contagious (contagious is not the same as infectious; although all contagious diseases are infectious, not all infectious diseases are contagious). These diseases can also be transmitted by sharing a towel (where the towel is rubbed vigorously on both bodies) or items of clothing in close contact with the body (socks, for example) if they are not washed thoroughly between uses. For this reason, contagious diseases often break out in schools, where towels are shared and personal items of clothing accidentally swapped in the changing rooms.

Some diseases that are transmissible by direct contact include athlete's foot, impetigo, syphilis (on rare occasions, if an uninfected person touches a chancre), warts, and conjunctivitis.[citation needed]

Droplet

"Droplet transmission occurs when respiratory droplets generated via coughing, sneezing or talking contact susceptible mucosal surfaces, such as the eyes, nose or mouth. Transmission may also occur indirectly via contact with contaminated formites with hands and then mucosal surfaces. Respiratory droplets are large and are not able to remain suspended in the air thus they are usually dispersed over short distances."[8]

The pathogen-containing particles, also called Flügge

droplets (after Carl Flügge), are 0,1–2 mm in diameter, and are reduced by evaporation to droplet nuclei – small (smaller than 100 μ in diameter), dry particles that can remain airborne for long periods.[9]

Organisms spread by droplet transmission include respiratory viruses (e.g., influenza, parainfluenza virus, adenovirus, respiratory syncytial virus, human metapneumovirus), Bordetella pertussis, pneumococci, diphtheria, and rubella.[10]

Fecal–oral

Main article: Fecal–oral route

In the fecal-oral route, pathogens in fecal particles pass from one person to the mouth of another person. Main causes of fecal–oral disease transmission include lack of adequate sanitation and poor hygiene practices - which can take various forms.

Fecal oral transmission can be via foodstuffs or water that has become contaminated. This can happen when people do not adequately wash their hands after using the toilet and before preparing food or tending to patients.

The fecal-oral route of transmission can be a public health risk for people in developing countries who live in urban slums without access to adequate sanitation. Here, excreta or untreated sewage can pollute drinking water sources (groundwater or surface water). The people who drink the polluted water can become infected. Another problem in some developing countries, such as India, is open defecation which leads to disease transmission via the fecal-oral route. Even in developed countries there are periodic system failures resulting in a sanitary sewer overflow. This is the typical mode of transmission for the infectious agents of for example: cholera, hepatitis A, polio, Rotavirus, Salmonella, and parasites (e.g. Ascaris lumbricoides).

RELATED SOURCES

https://en.wikipedia.org/wiki/Transmission_(medicine)

AVOIDING "OVERCROWDING"

Infectious disease during an emergency condition can raise the death rate 60 times in comparison to other causes including trauma. An epidemic, or outbreak, can occur when several aspects of the agent (pathogen), population (hosts), and the environment create an ideal situation for spread. Overcrowding, poor regional design and hygiene due to poverty, dirty drinking water, rapid climate changes, and natural disasters, can lead to conditions that allow easier transmission of disease. Once it has been established that an emergency condition exists, there must be a prompt and thorough response for communicable disease control. A camp should be created, and the disease managed rapidly. The overall goals are rapid assessment, prevention, surveillance, outbreak control, and disease management.

RELATED SOURCES

https://www.ncbi.nlm.nih.gov/pmc/articles/PMC4910139/

SUPERVISION OF "FOOD INTAKE"
Food safety *Key facts* *Access to sufficient amounts of safe and nutritious food is key to sustaining life and promoting good health.* *Unsafe food containing harmful bacteria, viruses, parasites or chemical substances, causes more than 200 diseases – ranging from diarrhoea to cancers.* *An estimated 600 million – almost 1 in 10 people in the world – fall ill after eating contaminated food and 420 000 die every year, resulting in the loss of 33 million healthy life years (DALYs).* *Children under 5 years of age carry 40% of the foodborne disease burden, with 125 000 deaths every year.* *Diarrhoeal diseases are the most common illnesses resulting from the consumption of contaminated food, causing 550 million people to fall ill and 230 000 deaths every year.* *Food safety, nutrition and food security are inextricably linked. Unsafe food creates a vicious cycle of disease and malnutrition, particularly affecting infants, young children, elderly and the sick.* *Foodborne diseases impede socioeconomic development by straining health care systems, and harming national economies, tourism and trade.* *Food supply chains now cross multiple national borders. Good collaboration between governments, producers and consumers helps ensure food safety.* *Major foodborne illnesses and causes* *Foodborne illnesses are usually infectious or toxic in*

nature and caused by bacteria, viruses, parasites or chemical substances entering the body through contaminated food or water.
Foodborne pathogens can cause severe diarrhoea or debilitating infections including meningitis.
Chemical contamination can lead to acute poisoning or long-term diseases, such as cancer. Foodborne diseases may lead to long-lasting disability and death.
Examples of unsafe food include uncooked foods of animal origin, fruits and vegetables contaminated with faeces, and raw shellfish containing marine biotoxins.
Bacteria:
Salmonella, Campylobacter, and Enterohaemorrhagic Escherichia coli are among the most common foodborne pathogens that affect millions of people annually – sometimes with severe and fatal outcomes. Symptoms are fever, headache, nausea, vomiting, abdominal pain and diarrhoea. Examples of foods involved in outbreaks of salmonellosis are eggs, poultry and other products of animal origin.
Foodborne cases with Campylobacter are mainly caused by raw milk, raw or undercooked poultry and drinking water. Enterohaemorrhagic Escherichia coli is associated with unpasteurized milk, undercooked meat and fresh fruits and vegetables.
Listeria infection leads to unplanned abortions in pregnant women or death of newborn babies. Although disease occurrence is relatively low, listeria's severe and sometimes fatal health consequences, particularly among infants, children and the elderly, count them among the most serious foodborne infections. Listeria is found in unpasteurised dairy products and various ready-to-eat foods and can grow at refrigeration temperatures.

Vibrio cholerae infects people through contaminated water or food. Symptoms include abdominal pain, vomiting and profuse watery diarrhoea, which may lead to severe dehydration and possibly death. Rice, vegetables, millet gruel and various types of seafood have been implicated in cholera outbreaks.
Antimicrobials, such as antibiotics, are essential to treat infections caused by bacteria. However, their overuse and misuse in veterinary and human medicine has been linked to the emergence and spread of resistant bacteria, rendering the treatment of infectious diseases ineffective in animals and humans. Resistant bacteria enter the food chain through the animals (e.g. Salmonella through chickens). Antimicrobial resistance is one of the main threats to modern medicine.
Viruses:
Norovirus infections are characterized by nausea, explosive vomiting, watery diarrhoea and abdominal pain. Hepatitis A virus can cause long-lasting liver disease and spreads typically through raw or undercooked seafood or contaminated raw produce. Infected food handlers are often the source of food contamination.
Parasites:
Some parasites, such as fish-borne trematodes, are only transmitted through food. Others, for example tapeworms like Echinococcus spp, or Taenia solium, may infect people through food or direct contact with animals. Other parasites, such as Ascaris, Cryptosporidium, Entamoeba histolytica or Giardia, enter the food chain via water or soil and can contaminate fresh produce.
Prions:

Prions, infectious agents composed of protein, are unique in that they are associated with specific forms of neurodegenerative disease. Bovine spongiform encephalopathy (BSE, or "mad cow disease") is a prion disease in cattle, associated with the variant Creutzfeldt-Jakob Disease (vCJD) in humans. Consuming bovine products containing specified risk material, e.g. brain tissue, is the most likely route of transmission of the prion agent to humans.
Chemicals:
Of most concern for health are naturally occurring toxins and environmental pollutants.
Naturally occurring toxins include mycotoxins, marine biotoxins, cyanogenic glycosides and toxins occurring in poisonous mushrooms. Staple foods like corn or cereals can contain high levels of mycotoxins, such as aflatoxin and ochratoxin, produced by mould on grain. A long-term exposure can affect the immune system and normal development, or cause cancer.
Persistent organic pollutants (POPs) are compounds that accumulate in the environment and human body. Known examples are dioxins and polychlorinated biphenyls (PCBs), which are unwanted by-products of industrial processes and waste incineration. They are found worldwide in the environment and accumulate in animal food chains. Dioxins are highly toxic and can cause reproductive and developmental problems, damage the immune system, interfere with hormones and cause cancer.
Heavy metalssuch as lead, cadmium and mercury cause neurological and kidney damage.
Contamination by heavy metal in food occurs mainly through pollution of air, water and soil.
The burden of foodborne diseases

The burden of foodborne diseases to public health and welfare and to economy has often been underestimated due to underreporting and difficulty to establish causal relationships between food contamination and resulting illness or death.

The 2015 WHO report on the estimates of the global burden of foodborne diseases presented the first-ever estimates of disease burden caused by 31 foodborne agents (bacteria, viruses, parasites, toxins and chemicals) at global and regional level.
WHO estimates of the global burden of foodborne diseases
The evolving world and food safety
Safe food supplies support national economies, trade and tourism, contribute to food and nutrition security, and underpin sustainable development.
Urbanization and changes in consumer habits, including travel, have increased the number of people buying and eating food prepared in public places.
Globalization has triggered growing consumer demand for a wider variety of foods, resulting in an increasingly complex and longer global food chain.
As the world's population grows, the intensification and industrialization of agriculture and animal production to meet increasing demand for food creates both opportunities and challenges for food safety.
Climate change is also predicted to impact food safety, where temperature changes modify food safety risks associated with food production, storage and distribution.
These challenges put greater responsibility on food producers and handlers to ensure food safety. Local incidents can quickly evolve into international

emergencies due to the speed and range of product distribution. Serious foodborne disease outbreaks have occurred on every continent in the past decade, often amplified by globalized trade.
Examples include the contamination of infant formula with melamine in 2008 (affecting 300 000 infants and young children, 6 of whom died, in China alone), and the 2011 Enterohaemorrhagic Escherichia coli outbreak in Germany linked to contaminated fenugreek sprouts, where cases were reported in 8 countries in Europe and North America, leading to 53 deaths and significant economic losses.
Food safety: a public health priority
Unsafe food poses global health threats, endangering everyone. Infants, young children, pregnant women, the elderly and those with an underlying illness are particularly vulnerable. Every year 220 million children contract diarrhoeal diseases and 96 000 die. Unsafe food creates a vicious cycle of diarrhoea and malnutrition, threatening the nutritional status of the most vulnerable. Where food supplies are insecure, people tend to shift to less healthy diets and consume more "unsafe foods" – in which chemical, microbiological and other hazards pose health risks.
The Second International Conference on Nutrition (ICN2), held in Rome in November 2014, reiterated the importance of food safety in achieving better human nutrition through healthy nutritious diets. Improving food safety is thus a key in achieving Sustainable Development Goals. Governments should make food safety a public health priority, as they play a pivotal role in developing policies and regulatory frameworks, establishing and implementing effective food safety systems that ensure that food producers

and suppliers along the whole food chain operate responsibly and supply safe food to consumers.
Food can become contaminated at any point of production and distribution, and the primary responsibility lies with food producers. Yet a large proportion of foodborne disease incidents are caused by foods improperly prepared or mishandled at home, in food service establishments or markets. Not all food handlers and consumers understand the roles they must play, such as adopting basic hygienic practices when buying, selling and preparing food to protect their health and that of the wider community.
Everyone can contribute to making food safe. Here are some examples of effective actions:

Policy-makers can:
build and maintain adequate food systems and infrastructures (e.g. laboratories) to respond to and manage food safety risks along the entire food chain, including during emergencies;
foster multi-sectoral collaboration among public health, animal health, agriculture and other sectors for better communication and joint action;
integrate food safety into broader food policies and programmes (e.g. nutrition and food security);
think globally and act locally to ensure the food produce domestically be safe internationally.
Food handlers and consumers can:
know the food they use (read labels on food package, make an informed choice, become familiar with common food hazards);
handle and prepare food safely, practicing the WHO Five Keys to Safer Food at home, or when selling at restaurants or at local markets;

grow fruits and vegetables using the WHO Five Keys to Growing Safer Fruits and Vegetables to decrease microbial contamination.

WHO response

WHO aims to facilitate global prevention, detection and response to public health threats associated with unsafe food. Ensuring consumer trust in their authorities, and confidence in the safe food supply, is an outcome that WHO works to achieve.

To do this, WHO helps Member States build capacity to prevent, detect and manage foodborne risks by:

providing independent scientific assessments on microbiological and chemical hazards that form the basis for international food standards, guidelines and recommendations, known as the Codex Alimentarius, to ensure food is safe wherever it originates;

assessing the safety of new technologies used in food production, such as genetic modification and nanotechnology;

helping improve national food systems and legal frameworks, and implement adequate infrastructure to manage food safety risks. The International Food Safety Authorities Network (INFOSAN) was developed by WHO and the UN Food and Agriculture Organization (FAO) to rapidly share information during food safety emergencies;

promoting safe food handling through systematic disease prevention and awareness programmes, through the WHO Five Keys to Safer Food message and training materials; and

advocating for food safety as an important component of health security and for integrating food safety into national policies and programmes in line with the International Health Regulations (IHR - 2005).

WHO works closely with FAO, the World Organization for Animal Health (OIE) and other international organizations to ensure food safety along the entire food chain from production to consumption.

Related

Fact sheets on food safety

WHO estimates of the global burden of foodborne diseases

Advancing Food Safety Initiatives

WHO strategic plan for food safety 2013-2022

WHO's work on food safety

RELATED SOURCES

https://www.who.int/news-room/fact-sheets/detail/food-safety

PROVIDING "BARRIER NURSING"

1. Barrier Nursing and Infection Control By Dr.(Mrs.)S.Valliammal College of Nursing NIMHANS Bangalore
2. Barrier Nursing &Infection ControlIntroduction The nursing technique by which a patient with an infectious disease is prevented from infecting other people is called barrier nursing
3. Hand hygiene is the simplest, most effective measure for infection control
4. Types of Precautions - BarrierNursing1. Contact Precautions2. Airborne Precautions3. Droplet Precautions4. Three more elements have been added to standard precautions. They are: 4.1 Respiratory hygiene/cough etiquette 4.2 Safe injection practices 4.3Use of masks for insertion of catheters or injection into spinal or epidural areas 4
5. 1. Contact Precautions□ Clean, non-sterile gloves are usually adequate for routine care of the patients□ Use gloves before providing care to patient Contd.....
6. □ Change gloves after contact with infective material.□ After providing care, remove gloves and wash hands□ Follow proper use of protective gown in case of direct contact with patient with potentially contaminated environmental surfaces and observe hand hygiene Contd....
7. □ Limit the movement or transport of the patient from the room.□ Make sure any infected or colonized areas are contained or covered.□ Ensure that patient care items, bedside equipment and frequently touched surfaces receive daily cleaning. 7
8. 2. Airborne Precautions□ Used to prevent or reduce

the transmission of micro-organisms that are airborne in small droplet nuclei (5 or smaller in size) or dust particles containing the infectious agent. Contd.....
9. □ Place the patient in private room that has negative air pressure, with 6-12 air changes/per hour.□ If not available, cohort with patient with active infection with same microorganism□ Use of respiratory protection Contd.....
10. □ Limit movement and transport of the patient.□ Use a mask on the patient if they need to be moved□ Keep patient room door closed.
11. 3. Droplet Precautions□ Used to reduce the risk of transmission of microorganisms transmitted by large particle droplets (larger than 5 in size).□ Droplets usually travel 3 feet or less within the air and thus special air handling is not required, however newer recommendations suggest a distance of 6 feet be used for safety. Contd....
12. □ Place the patient in a private room□ Use of respiratory protection such as a mask when entering the room recommended and definitely if within 3 feet of patient□ Limit movement and transport of the patient Contd....
13. □ Use a mask on the patient if they need to be moved and follow respiratory hygiene/cough etiquette□ Keep patient at least 3 feet apart between infected patient and visitors□ Room door may remain open
14. 4.1 Respiratory Hygiene/Cough Etiquette• Informing personnel if they have any symptoms of respiratory infection• Health educate patients and visitors to cover their mouth/nose while coughing and sneezing Contd......
15. • Proper disposal of used materials, during coughing and sneezing• Use of surgical masks on

coughing person when appropriate• Providing alcohol-based hand-rubbing dispensers and supplies for hand hygiene and educating patients and staff in their use,• Encouraging hand hygiene after coughing or sneezing. Contd....

16. • Separating coughing persons at least 3 feet away from others in a waiting room or have separate locality.• Instructing patients and providers not to touch eyes, nose, or mouth.• Health care workers should use standard precautions with all patients. Contd....

17. 4.2 Safe injection practices • Correct disposal in appropriate container • Avoid re-sheathing needle • Avoid removing needle • Discard syringes as single unit • Avoid over-filling sharps container

18. 4.3 Use of masks for insertion ofcatheters or injection into spinalor epidural areas 18

19. Barrier Techniques Infection Control1. Aseptic technique2. Isolation3. Safer Handling of Sharps4. Linen handling and disposal5. Waste disposal6. Handling Biological Spills7. Environmental cleaning8. Risk assessment9. Staff health

*20. Barrier Techniques Infection Control1. Aseptic technique ◦ Medical Asepsis – Clean technique; procedures used to reduce & prevent spread of microorganisms ** Hand washing** ◦ Surgical Asepsis – Sterile technique; procedures used to eliminate microorganisms **Sterilization** Contd....*

21. 2. Isolation□ Source or protective□ Source - isolation of infected patient ◦ mainly to prevent airborne transmission via respiratory droplets ◦ Patients with SARS, pulmonary tuberculosis etc□ Protective - isolation of immune-suppressed patient Contd...

22. 3. Safer Handling of Sharps□ Prevention Aspects - Handle with much care - correct disposal in appropriate container□ Management ◦ follow hospital policy Contd...

23. 4. Linen handling and disposal□ Bed making and linen changing techniques□ Appropriate laundry bags□ Hazards of on-site ward-based laundering Contd.....

24. 5.Waste disposal□ Clinical waste - HIGH risk ◦ potentially/actually contaminated waste including body fluids and human tissue ◦ yellow plastic sack, tied prior to incineration□ Follow hospital policy Contd......

25. 6. Handling Biological Spills□ Cover area with hypochlorite solution for several minutes□ Clean area with warm water and detergent, then dry□ Treat waste as clinical waste - yellow plastic sack□ Follow hospital policy Contd...

26. 7. Environmental cleaning"Hospitals should do the sick no harm" (Nightingale, 1854) A study conducted by Moore etal ,2011- High touched sites in an hospital environment□ Bedside rails: 100%□ Blood pressure cuff: 88 'High-touch sites'□ Bedside Table: 63%□ Toilets: 63%

27. 8.Risk assessment□ No risk - routine care□ Low or moderate risk - wear gloves and plastic apron□ High risk (Contact/splashing) - wear gloves, plastic apron, gown, eye/face protection Contd....

28. 9.Staff health□ Risk of acquiring and transmitting infection□ Acquiring infection ◦ immunisation ◦ cover lesions with waterproof dressings ◦ restrict non-immune/pregnant staff□ Transmitting infection ◦ advice when suffering infection□ Report accidents/untoward incidents□ Follow hospital policy Contd.... 28

29. Staff health - Hand Care□ Nails□ Rings□ Hand creams□ Cuts & abrasions□ "Chapping"□ Skin Problems

30. Successful Promotion □ Infection control□

Continuous Nursing Education programme Routine observation & feedback Engineering controls ◦ Location of hand basins ◦ Possible, easy & convenient ◦ Alcohol-based hand rubs Patient education Contd...
31. Successful Promotion Reminders in the workplace Promote and facilitate skin care Avoid understaffing and excessive workload
33. Core references Davies, H. and Rees, J. (2000) Psychological effects of isolation nursing (1): mood disturbance. Nursing Standard. 14, 28, 35-38. May, D. (2000) Infection control. Nursing Standard. 14, 28. 51-57. ICNA (1998) Guidelines for hand hygiene. Belper: ICNA. NHS Executive (1995) Hospital laundry arrangements for used and infected linen - HSG (95) 18. London: DoH. Nightingale, F. (1854) Notes on nursing. Edinburgh: Churchill Livingstone
34. Internet sites http://www.icna.co.uk/
http://www.nursing-standard.co.uk/
http://www.medscape.com/
http://www.anes.uab.edu/medhist.htm
http://www.shef.ac.uk/~nhcon/
http://medweb.bham.ac.uk/nursing/
http://www.healthcentre.org.uk/hc/library/defa ult.htm
34
Recommended
Jean-Baptiste Dumont
AI and Machine Learning Demystified by Carol Smith at Midwest UX 2017
AI and Machine Learning Demystified by Carol Smith at Midwest UX 2017

RELATED SOURCES

https://www.slideshare.net/Valliammal2013/drsvalliammal-barrier-nursing-infection-control

RESTRICTION OF MOVEMENT OF "TRAVELLERS"
Much research in epidemiology has been focused on evaluating conventional methods of control strategies in the event of an epidemic or pandemic. Travel restrictions are often suggested as an efficient way to reduce the spread of a contagious disease that threatens public health, but few papers have studied in depth the effects of travel restrictions. In this study, we investigated what effect different levels of travel restrictions might have on the speed and geographical spread of an outbreak of a disease similar to severe acute respiratory syndrome (SARS). ***RELATED SOURCES*** *https://www.slideshare.net/Valliammal2013/drsvalliammal-barrier-nursing-infection-control*

DESCRIPTION OF THE MACHINE
Lingual-Numeric Calculator Definition It is a three-dimensional formula that was designed to complement the work of modern computer in a way that is direct and precise for the advancement of human knowledge. It supports the Pythagorean assertion which says: "All things had their origin and composition in numbers". It was allegorically expressed as: First Dimension Input= [OI x Q] A Slide per Letter Output In Figures=Cardinal Value Second Dimension Input=[1] + [OI x Q] A Slide per Letter

Output In Figures =First Ordinal Value [or the first serial number]
Third Dimension
Input=[OI x P] A Slide per Letter
Output In Figures=Second Ordinal Value [or the second serial number]
Full Meaning Of The Abbreviations:
O-Stands for the overall number of English alphabets [26]
I-Stands for indexes (in descending order) to which the overall number of English alphabets will be multiply by itself. It depends on the number of letters inside a word
Q-Stands for the quantitative value of each letter of English when they are arranged in an alphabetic order
P-Stands for the position of each letter of English when they are arranged in an alphabetic order
For example:
The Quantitative Value Of Each Letter Of English
A=0,B=1,C=2,D=3,E=4,F=5,G=6,H=7,I=8,J=9,K=10,L=11,M=12
N=13,O=14,P=15,Q=16,R=17,S=18,T=19,U=20,V=21,W=22,X=23,Y=
Z=25
The Position Of Each Letter Of English
A=1,B=2,C=3,D=4,E=5,F=6,G=7,H=8,I=9,J=10,K=11,L=12,M=13N=14,O=15,
P=16,Q=17,R=18,S=19,T=20,U=21,V=22,W=23,X=24,Y=25,Z=25
Algorithm
-Input
Input can be any word of interest. It can be a name of disease, term, course, discipline etc
-Data

Data is the representation of `a word in accordance with the three components of the machine, namely: overall number, indexes and quantity

-Computing

Computing is the act of reading a word according to the computational system of the machine.

-Output

Output are two: in figures and in words:

-Output in figures is the cardinal or ordinal value of an input.

-Output in word are vocabularies or sentences recognized by the
machine during the process of interpretation of an input

Language Of The Machine:

The basic difference between computer and lingual-numeric calculator is the language of the machine: the former understands 0 & 1[mechanically: 'on' & 'off'], while the later understands1 & 1 [literally: 'relevant' or 'irrelevant' based on 'characters']

Mechanism Of Data Processing For An Output

Firstly, upon entering an input, the machine will ask you to select from one of the three dimensions of the formula. Secondly, it will derive an ordinal scale from the obtained value for segmented coding. Thirdly, the machine is going to compute the value obtained into the language of the machine for integrated coding. Fourthly, the machine will start working on various sets of database [e.g. f1, f2, f3, f4, etc] for output processing. It categorizes words into two supporting components, such as: vocabulary [one or more] and sentence [one or more].

Vocabulary- only the relevant words would be recognized by the machine, while the irrelevant words would not be recognized for lack of associated characters literally or metaphorically.

- Sentence- the machine would only recognize a sentence whose integrated code doesn't contradict the integrated code of the subject in a sentence and the general contents of the first component

Segmented Code:

Is the act of considering all the numbers inside the cardinal or ordinal value of an input when making interpretation, it always requires an ordinal scale.

Integrated Code:

Is the act of considering a number reduced into the language of the machine from the cardinal or ordinal value of an input when making interpretation. It can be dependent or independent.

For example-it is dependent when it was used to interpret an ordinal scale of other input, but it is independent when it was used to interpret itself.

Method Of Database Processing Used By The Machine:

F1=[1-letter word database]
F2=[2-letter word database]
F3=[3-letter word database]
F4=[4-letter word database]
F5=[5-letter word database] up to F22=[22-letter word database]

Hence, any word with more than 22 letters would be read as coined word whose morphemes will be computed separately, before joining into one word.

SOURCE

Rahali lawali: lingual –numeric calculator